Hair Thinning!!

The Simple Truth

By: Iris Trussell

Licensed Cosmetologist

Table of Content

Inspiration

Being in the profession of cosmetology, I have serviced many clients who were suffering from problems associated with hair thinning or hair damage. In addition to these problems come stress, lack of self-esteem, and hormone issues, to name a few. I always try to give some encouragement along the way and give tips on how to care for the hair.

Sometimes you may feel down because your hair is not in a healthy state which doesn't do much for your self-esteem. But if your hair is healthy and neatly groomed, it can be the bridge that makes you get up and feel better about yourself.

I was not always on top of my game. There was a time when I first had children and the stress of being a young mother as well as a wife took a toll on me. I realized that I had to do better when I looked back at some pictures of myself that were taken some years prior. I didn't like what I saw. I had let myself go and didn't realize it. Then I began to wonder why it seemed that there was not as much physical attraction in my relationship as there once were. Then it hit me! I had to be honest with myself. If I looked like this to him, no wonder some attraction was gone.

What I am saying is that its time to pick yourself up. It's not too late to turn things around. GET UP! And GET OUT OF THE HOUSE!! Go to the mall and get a make over. Go to a licensed hairstylist and let them give you a style that fits you.

Your life begins when you say and take the initiative. Get a manicure!! Get a massage!! You don't have to pay a fortune. There are students at your local cosmetology and massage therapy school, training under a licensed instructor, who can give you a massage, manicure, hairstyle or makeover for half the cost of a professional salon.

But if you can afford a professional, you owe it to yourself. When I first attended cosmetology school, I looked around and I saw all the students that were juniors and seniors looking professional and well groomed. Hairstyles that brought out their best features, sculptured nails with nail art, and make-up that pulled everything together. I then realized that I wanted to look like that. Then my mission began.

Get Up! Get It Together!!

Acknowledgements

I would like to first thank God who is the head of my life. I have been through many tests, trials, and tribulations, yet I'm still here. I would like to thank my husband, Gerrnero, who stayed in the tests, trials, and tribulations with me who also had tests of his own, and who has grown in the Lord by trust and faith. I would like to thank our sons, Gerrnero Jr., Jeremy, and Jamari, who have been my comedy and entertainment. Thanks for being great kids. I Love You.

I thank God for my grandparents, Jessie and Alice Williams (deceased), who gave me my morals, foundation, taught me to have respect for my elders, and to love everybody. A special thanks to my mother, Mary Fountain, whom I have watched over the years, go for what she wanted and never stopped until accomplishing her goals in life. I know that I got that from her. I must send a shout out to my sisters, Taundra and Ashley (Nae Nae), Fountain, whom I had lots of laughs and fun times with over the years. Thanks to my niece, Amia Lewis, "my other child", whom I share a special bond with. I Love you. To my Step Father, Kenneth Fountain, whom I was blessed with and still hold very fond memories of as a child coming to the country, fixing my bike, and playing with me. Thanks. To my dad, Dove Hall, whom I received the "gift of lecturing," and my kids just love that. I give you thanks. I give many thanks to Shirley Williams, my aunt, who was my spiritual advisor early in marriage. If it were not for you, we might not have made it. Thanks also for critiquing this book. May God bless you! I thank Hattie Mae, my aunt, who was like a mother to me. Thanks for being there. To

Cathryn Hall, "Grandma Cathryn," who always has a listening ear and encourages me in every way. I give you thanks and I love you. To my sisters, Shirley Gardner and Unique Hankston, I am grateful for both of you. To my brothers Jovantia Johnson and Ethan L Hall, I am thankful for you. To my aunts Jessie Mable and Bertha (deceased), Mary Helen, Arnell, Sadie, Lillie Belle and Geraldine and uncles, James (tac), Dan Henry (DH) and Rev. Carl Williams, Thanks for being an important influence in my life. To Mr. and Mrs. Sam & Odie Green who are great grandparents to our kids. I also want to thank you for being there for me when I needed it the most.

Last, but not least, thanks to my Pastor Ronald L. Patton, who is truly a man of God. I also want to thank his wife, Nedra Patton for being there to offer her support. Thank you for your prayers, advice, love and genuine care for my family and me.

Finally, thanks to my instructors: Robert Kirkland, Nancy Black, Reba Roy, Shirley Little, Mable Ross, Elizabeth Williams, Flora Johnson and Tony Brown. Without all of you, I never would have made it.

Helpful Spiritual Scriptures

Galatians 5: 22-23

But the Holy Spirit produces this kind of fruit in our lives: love, joy, peace, patience, kindness, goodness, faithfulness, gentleness and self-control. There is no Law against these things.

1 Corinthians 11:15

And isn't long hair a woman's pride and joy? For it has been given to her as a covering.

1 Timothy 2:9

And I want women to be modest in their appearance(or to pray in modest apparel) they should wear decent and appropriate clothing and not draw attention to themselves by the way they fix their hair, or by wearing gold or pearls or expensive clothes.

1 Peter 3:3

Don't be concerned about the outward beauty of fancy hairstyles, expensive jewelry or beautiful clothes.

Matthew 6:7

But when you fast, comb your hair and wash your face.

Psalms 45:11

For your royal husband delights in your beauty; honor him, for he is your lord.

Proverbs 16:31

Gray hair is a crown of Glory; it is gained by living a Godly life.

Proverbs 31:30

Charm is deceptive and beauty does not last; but a woman who fears the lord will be greatly praised.

1 Peter 3:4

You should clothe yourselves instead with the beauty that comes from within; the unfading beauty of a gentle and quiet spirit which is so precious to God.

James 1:5

If any of you lacks wisdom, He should ask God, who gives generously to all without finding fault, and it will be given to him.

John 3:16

For God so loved the world that he gave his only begotten son, that whosoever believeth in him shall not parish but have everlasting life.

Composition of Hair

Before we get started, there are some things you must know about the composition or structure of hair. First, hair is made up chiefly of a protein called Keratin and consists of three layers: The Cuticle, Cortex and Medulla.

The Cuticle is the outer most layer and is made up of transparent, overlapping horny scale-like cells that protect the inner layers of the hair.

The Cortex is the inner or middle layer which is where the strength and elasticity (the ability to stretch and return back to its original shape without breaking) is housed. This layer is where chemical changes (Relaxers, Permanent waves, and permanent hair- coloring, etc.) takes place and is where the melanin (pigment or color) is located which gives hair its color.

The inner most layer is called the Medulla, also referred to as the pith or marrow. There is no known function of this layer. The medulla may be absent from fine or very fine hair.

Now that you have learned about the composition and layers of hair, you need to understand the main parts in which hair is divided. The first part is the Hair Root, which is found beneath or under the scalp or skin. The second part is the Hair Shaft (Strand) which is above or comes out of the scalp. Hair is not a living tissue. It does not contain any nerves and is not sensitive to pain when being cut. Hair is cells that are not living anymore. The living tissue is the hair root which is underneath the skin and is nourished through the blood supply.

Understanding the Hair Root

There are also structures associated with the hair root. They are the Hair Follicle, Hair bulb and the Papilla. The Hair follicle, in simple terms, is the hole that the hair comes out of. This hole encases the hair root and every hair has its own follicle. The Hair Bulb is a thickened, club-shaped structure forming the lower part of the hair root where hair growth begins. The lower part of the hair bulb is hollow and it fits over the hair papilla. The Papilla is a small cone-shaped elevation at the bottom of the hair follicle that fits into the hair bulb. In the papilla is a rich blood and nerve supply, which contributes to the growth and regeneration of the hair. Nourishment reaches the hair bulb through the papilla. If the papilla is well nourished and healthy, it will produce hair cells

that will cause new hair to grow. If the papilla is
destroyed, the hair will not grow.

Hair Structure

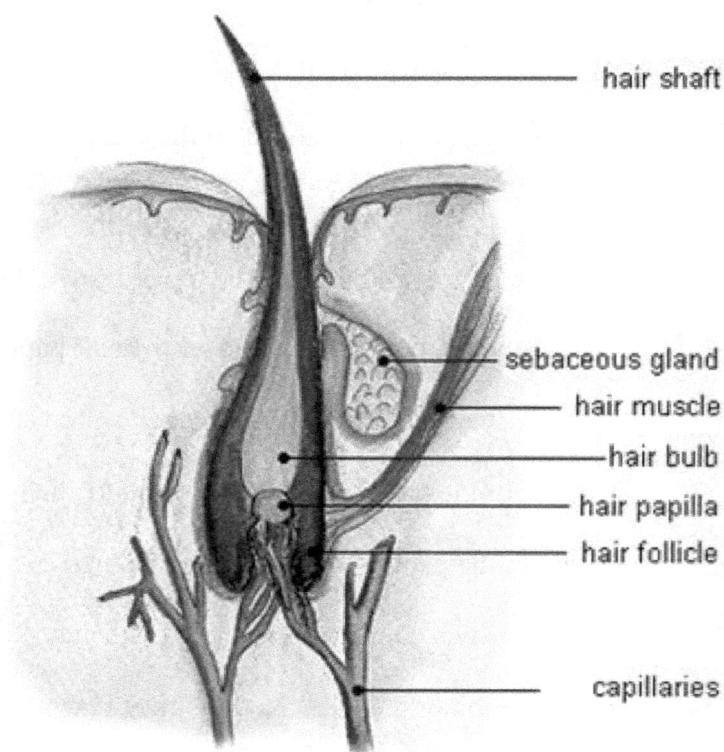

hair shaft

sebaceous gland

hair muscle

hair bulb

hair papilla

hair follicle

capillaries

Hair structure by: becomehealthynow.com

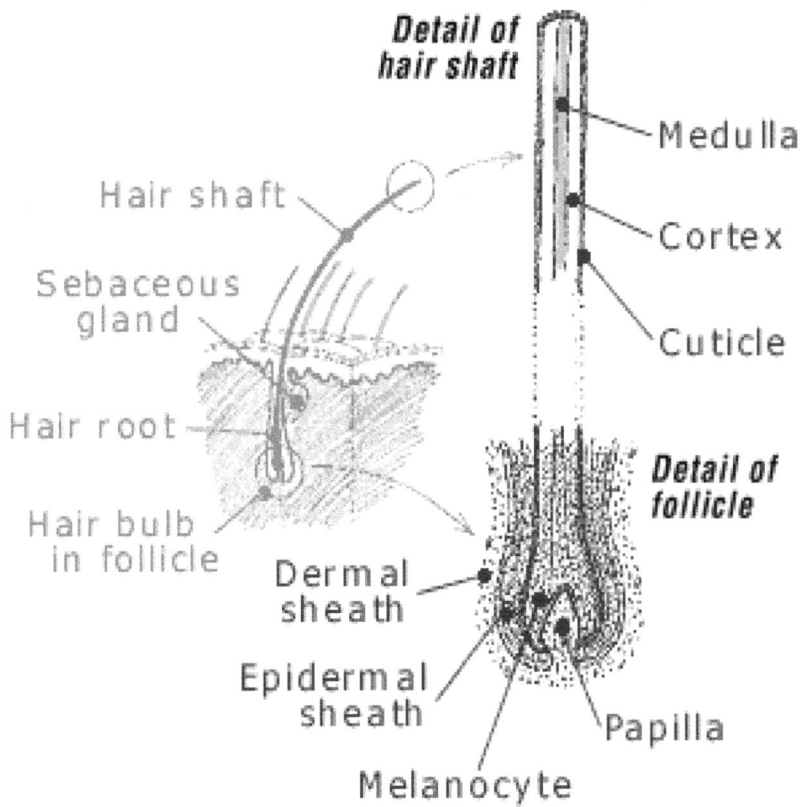

Diagram by: exploratorium.edu

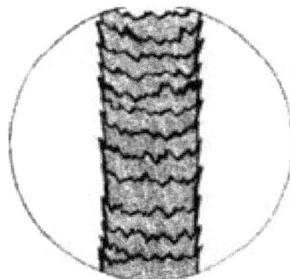

Cuticle layer.   Diagram by: haircoloringtip.net

Why am I telling you this?

In order to understand how to care for your hair, you must first understand the hair itself. If you know that hair grows through the blood and nerve supply, then you must realize that you must have a healthy blood supply and diet that promotes growth.

Many people go on crash diets or diets that cut out or cut down protein. Big Mistake! In an earlier chapter, you learned that hair is composed chiefly of a Protein called Keratin. That being said, if you take away all protein then you are taking away the nutrient that the hair is made of. That's not to say go on a protein quest, but make sure you eat well balanced meals. Consult your physician for help with a balanced diet.

Hair Growth

When the hair is healthy and normal, hair strands go through cycles: growth, fall and replacement. The formation and the growth of hair cells depend on proper nourishment and oxygen which can only be supplied by the bloodstream. Therefore, blood is essential to the healthiness and life of the hair. On average, hair grows about ½ inches per month. The normal growth cycle is 2 to 6 years and accounts for about 90 percent of the hair strand's life cycle. Hair growth starts in the papilla. If the papilla is destroyed, the hair will not grow. New hair is formed by cell division from a growing point at the root around the papilla.

When the hair is in the fall phase, the bulb loosens and separates from the papilla. Then the bulb moves upward in the follicle. Finally, the hair moves slowly to the surface, where it is shed. In normal hair shed, 75 to 150 strands of hair may be shed per day. If there is shedding of more than this, it may indicate a problem. See a physician.

The last cycle is replacement, or resting phase, which may last for several weeks. All growth has ceased and the bulb has weakened at the level of the sebaceous canal. As the hair fiber rests prior to shedding, new hair growth begins and the cycle is completed.

It is absolutely necessary to get regular hair trims. This will help to keep your hair healthy and free from split ends. Once the hair has split ends, the damage will continue to work its way up the hair strands until the hair is cut beyond the damage. As a general rule of thumb, I usually trim at each relaxer or as needed, based on the condition of the hair. That's about every five to six weeks.

Factors That May Affect Hair Growth

Diet

Medication, Drugs and Illnesses

Scalp Disorders/Abnormalities and Heredity

Stress, Hormones, Giving Birth

Misuse of Products, Implements or Tools

Diet

As stated earlier, it is not a good idea to go on a crash diet. The body, as well as the hair needs a balanced diet. When you deprive the body of important vitamins and nutrients, your whole body, not only your hair reacts to the deficiency. You may experience tiredness, weakness, depression, headaches, dizziness, cramps, and slothfulness etc., without the proper diet. Important vitamins such as A, C, E and D are important in the growth of hair, skin and nails. Ask your physician about a balanced diet that is right for you.

Medications/Drugs and Illnesses

Since the hair gets its nourishment through the blood supply, it is safe to say that if the blood is not healthy then the growth will not be at its fullest potential. Some illnesses or drugs may be a factor in hair thinning.

According to WebMD and Mary Sheen's, Fighting Hair Loss, the following is a list of drugs known for hair thinning.

Illness	Drugs
Acne	Accutane (Isotretinoin) and Tegison(etretinate) drugs derived from Vitamin-A
Blood	Anticoagulants-(blood thinners), Panwarfin, Sofarin, Coumadin, Heparin Injections
Cholesterol	Atromid-S (clofibrate), Lopid (gemfibrozil)
Convulsions/ Epilepsy	Anticonvulsants- Trimethadione (Tridione)
Depression	Antidepressants- Anafranil(clomipramine), Elavil(amitriptyline), Paxil, Pamelor, Prozac, Tofranil, Zoloft, Sinequan
Diet	Amphetamines(weight loss)

Fungus	Antifungals
Glaucoma	Beta-blocker drugs, including Timoptic Eye Drops(timolol) Timoptic Ocudose, Timoptic XE
Gout	Zyloprim(allopurinol)
Heart/High Blood Pressure	Including Beta-blockers, Tenormin (atenolol), Metoprolol (lopressor), Corgard (nadolol), Inderal/Inderal LA (propranolol), Blocadren (timolol)
Hormonal Conditions	Birth control pills, Hormone-replacement therapy(HRT) for women(estrogen/progestrone) Male androgenic hormones
Hormonal	all forms of testosterone

Hormonal conditions cont.	Anabolic steroids, Prednisone and other steroids
Inflammation, Arthritis	Nonsteroidal anti-inflammatory drugs including: Naprosyn(naproxen), Anaprox(naproxen), Anaprox DS(naproxen), Indocin(indomethacin) Indocin SR(indomethacin), Clinoril(sulindac), Penicillamine, Ridaura(auranofin), Folex *Methotrexate(MTX) and *Rheumatrex .
Parkinson's Disease	Levadopa/L-dopa (Dopar, Laradopa)

Thyroid Disorders	Carbimazole, Iodine, Thiocyanate, Thiouracil
Ulcer	Tagament(cimetidine) Zantac(ranitidine), Pepcid(famotidine

*also used as chemotherapy drug

Ask your physician if there is an alternative if you are on medications for any of these illnesses.

Abnormal Scalp Disorders and Heredity

There are many scalp disorders or abnormal scalp conditions that may retard or slow down hair growth. Some may be hereditary. There are quite a few problems that are passed down through genes. If your parents have hair loss or thinning, then there is a great chance that their children will have the same issues with thinning. The more people in ones family with hair loss, the greater the chance they will inherit it. In my years of consulting with clients, I found that the number one problem associated with hair thinning is "itching". Almost all clients had this one issue in common. In this instance, one of the first things I advise the client to do is stop scratching. When you use your fingernails to scratch, you are causing irritation to the scalp. I recommend them to use scalp oil, usually tea tree oil, which has an anti-fungal agent that can sooth the scalp. I advise them that if they feel the need to scratch, use a brush or comb to satisfy the itch, instead of your nails. If you feel that you have a severe problem with hair thinning, a skin Biopsy or other procedures may be used to diagnose medical disorders that cause loss of hair. Some of the most common abnormal scalp conditions are: *Scaling, Dandruff, Inflammations, Psoriasis, Eczema, Cradle Cap, Seborrhea, Impetigo, Ringworm, and Alopecia.*

Scaling Conditions

Dandruff, scientifically called *Pityriasis Capitis,* is the presence of small, white scales on the scalp and hair, caused by the excessive shedding of the epithelial scales. Instead of growing to the surface and falling off, they accumulate on the scalp and may be caused by poor circulation, infection, injury, lack of nerve stimulation, improper diet or uncleanliness. In some instances, using strong shampoo's containing harsh soaps and not rinsing away products or allowing buildup of styling agents to accumulate on your scalp may add to the problem.

There are two main types of dandruff: *Dry dandruff and Greasy (waxy) dandruff.* Dry dandruff consists of an itchy scalp with small white scales that may be scattered loosely in the hair. This type sometimes falls to the shoulders. Dry dandruff can be treated with frequent shampooing using mild shampoos, scalp treatments or scalp antiseptics. Oil, specifically for itchy scalp may be useful as a daily scalp treatment. These usually contain some type of medication.

Greasy (waxy) dandruff, medically called *Pityriasis Steatoides*, is scaliness of the epidermis, mixed with sebum (oil) which causes it to stick to the scalp in patches. Bleeding or oozing may occur if these greasy scales are torn off. Seek medical treatment.

You must treat all dandruff as being contagious, therefore make sure to sanitize combs, brushes etc, and do not use or permit anyone to use your hair implements. There is no such thing as "growing dandruff".

Inflammations

Dermatitis is a general term for an inflammation of the skin. *Psoriasis* is a chronic inflammatory skin disease, of scaling or redness, which cause is unknown. If severe, it may lead to hair loss. Psoriasis is lesions that are round, dry patches covered with coarse, silvery scales. It can be found on the scalp, elbows, knees, chest and lower back, but rarely on the face. If irritated, bleeding may occur, but it is not contagious. Ointments, as well as other items are available to clear this skin disease.

Eczema is an inflammation of the skin that may be acute or chronic. The lesions may be dry or moist which may be followed by burning or itching. There is no known cause and all Eczema conditions should be referred to a physician. *Cradle cap*, in babies may be an early form of atopic eczema which is associated with hay fever and asthma or the mother's milk.

Seborrhea is another skin condition that may affect the scalp. This is a result of overactive or excessive secretion of the Sebaceous gland. Seborrhea on the scalp may cause the scalp to itch and show the presence of an unusual amount of oil on the hair. An oily or shiny nose or forehead may also indicate seborrhea.

Impetigo is a bacterial infection of the skin, resulting in crusted sores, itching and weeping. This is most often seen in young children and may affect the scalp and face. Impetigo must be referred to a physician for treatment.

Ringworm is a fungal infection which is recognized as round, pink and scaly patches with raised edges. Ringworm is highly contagious and must be treated by prescription by mouth. Ringworm spreads when hair implements are shared and when you touch the affected area and don't wash your hands immediately. Ringworm, if not treated immediately will cause hair loss that could be permanent.

Abnormal Hair Loss

Alopecia is the technical term for any abnormal hair loss. This is not natural loss of hair. Natural hair loss occurs when the hair is normal and healthy and each individual strand goes through a cycle of growth, fall and replacement. When hair has grown through its course, it comes out and is replaced by new hair. In alopecia, the hair does not come back unless special treatments are given which may encourage hair regrowth.

There are three common forms of alopecia. ***Alopecia Senilis, alopecia Areata and alopecia Prematura.*** *Alopecia Senilis* is baldness that occurs in old age. *Alopecia Areata* is baldness in spots or patches. This baldness could be caused by anemia, scarlet fever, typhoid fever or syphilis. The sight of alopecia areata may be smooth, shiny with very few or no hair follicles. Therefore, if there are no hair follicles, there will not be a production of hair unless there is treatment or hair replacement therapy. In a lot of cases, there has been some injury to the nervous system and since the flow of blood is influenced by the nervous system, the affected area is usually under nourished. In alopecia prematura, baldness occurs or starts before middle age such as in children. The process starts with a slow, thinning process where the hair that falls out is replaced with thinner or weaker strands.

Some treatments for alopecia are ultra-violet and infra-red therapy combined with the use of stimulating creams, shampoos, and conditioners as well as massaging of the scalp in the affected area.

Stress Related Hair Loss

Stress or "nerves" is a popular factor that is used a lot in today's society. With the changes in the economy, a rise in the cost of living, violence, personal problems in marriage, family and finances, we are suffering with more stress-related illnesses than ever before. Stress can alter the intake of certain trace elements and amino acids essential for hair growth. It is said to account for about 30% of hair loss in women but it can regrow if the nutritional deficiency is restored.

High levels of stress can increase levels of the hormone, prolactin in women and this appears to influence the increase of testosterone, which converts to DHT (Dihydrotestosterone) interrupting the hair growth cycle. To certain degrees, this can lead to hair thinning. DHT is the result of chemical imbalances and occurs in your blood stream. It builds up around the hair follicle and prevents the blood from reaching your hair follicle causing the hair follicle to be undernourished and slowly begin to die. As a result, the hair thins out and the hair follicles are minimized in size which, over time permanently kills the follicle altogether. For instance, you may see a person whose scalp is shiny and slick and there is no presence of hair follicles. The hair follicles have close completely as there is no more hair to keep them open. Androgenetic Alopecia is the main cause of this type of hair loss in both men and women.

Stress can also cause the arteries to narrow and restrict blood flow to the scalp, which means that hair loss, short term or permanent, may occur if there is not sufficient blood flow to the papilla. The first thing that I say to people with hair thinning problems is, "don't worry and stress over it, because it will only make matters worst". I know it is easier said than done.

Hair Loss after Pregnancy

The first instance that you know you are pregnant, start thinking about your hair. What I mean is pay attention to how you treat your hair. Make sure that you are eating properly, taking proper care and using the right products. The better the overall condition of the hair, the better luck you'll have maintaining it after you give birth. When you are pregnant, the hair usually doesn't shed as it would normally if you were not pregnant. The body will retain as much as it can for the baby. After birth, the body goes back to normal and a lot of time everything that didn't shed may shed at this time. Not everyone experiences excessive hair loss or thinning. Also, consider the fact of the epidural. This is the anesthesia used for pain during childbirth. This can also sometimes cause a loss of hair which is usually temporary. Between the second and seventh month after childbirth is usually when you will see hair loss. This is also likely to fluctuating levels in hormones. Sometimes continued use of pre-natal vitamins may help. In all situations, consult your physician.

Hair Loss Due to Misuse of Products or Implements

Sometimes you can contribute to your own hair loss by the misuse of products. Before you get excited about that popular new haircolor, or relaxer system, you must first understand the relationship between the hair and how the chemical works. At the beginning of this book, I gave important information about structures of the hair. Now you must also know about the different hair textures (degree of fineness or coarseness of hair) they are Fine, Medium and Coarse.

Fine or very fine texture requires special care. The medulla is missing in this hair texture. Only products specifically designed and formulated for this hair texture should be used. Using products for medium or coarse texture could cause extensive breakage, hair loss, or could cause the hair not to style as desired. If your hair doesn't hold well, or is lifeless, your products may be too heavy or too much product is being used. Follow the manufacturer's instructions when applying styling aids. Sometimes a nickel or quarter size amount is enough. Take the product and pour it in your hands, work it into your hands, then apply evenly through hair. Choose products with light hold or products that add volume to the hair. If you need to use heat appliances, purchase one with a temperature control, so you can adjust the level of heat. Fine hair usually calls for a low heat setting; otherwise hair can become quickly damaged by excessive heat. Also, make sure you use some type of protector prior to heat styling. If at all possible use Ceramic styling tools.

Ceramics are designed to heat the hair from inside

out not causing the hair to singe or burn on the outside. It is the healthier styling tool on the market. Texture does matter.

Medium texture is the most common type. The cortex, cuticle and medulla are all present but to a lesser degree. If your hair is not fine or coarse, this is more so, your hair texture. As with fine hair, use products designed and formulated for normal or medium textured hair. Styling tools are usually recommended on a medium setting and you tend to be able to take a little more heat. Use ceramics whenever possible.

Coarse hair also contains the cortex, cuticle and medulla. Coarse hair has the widest diameter. When dealing with coarse hair, it is more resistant than any other hair type. Therefore, it takes a stronger chemical to break the hair down or open the cuticle to perform a chemical service.

With that said, if you use a chemical designed for fine hair, the chemical will not be strong enough to break down the bonds of the hair and as a result, the hair will be under- processed. On the contrary, if you use a product too strong for your hair texture, it will result in being over- processed.

Strength of Products

The strength of a product is indicated on what is known as a pH scale. The pH scale (potential hydrogen) is used to show the degree of acidity of alkalinity. The pH scale ranges from 0-14. Each increase of one indicates an increase of acidity or alkalinity by ten-fold. The acidity or alkalinity of cosmetic or hair products influence the affect of the various layers of hair and or skin. Acidic products will shrink and harden and alkaline products soften, swell and expand the hair. Anything below 7.0 on the scale is acidic, and anything above 7.0 is alkaline. The higher the pH, the stronger the degree of alkalinity. The lower the pH the stronger the degree of acidity. 7.0 on the pH scale is distilled or pure water. Normal, healthy hair is 4.5-5.5. All chemical service solutions are alkaline. On the following pages, the approximate pH of various products and other items are listed. This pH scale may vary by manufacturers. This will give you a general idea about the strength of products used on your hair. Remember, the closer you are to 0 on the acidic side of the scale, the stronger the product. The closer you are to 14 on the alkaline side of the scale, the stronger the product.

pH Scale

pH	Substance	
0	Hydrochloric Acid	*strong acids*
0.5	Muriatic Acid	
2	Cream Rinses	
3	Dye Solvents	
3.5	Gels	
4	Hair Conditioner/Shampoo	
4.5-5.5	Normal Hair, skin	
5	Temporary Rinses	
6	Peroxide	*weak acids*
6.5	Permanent Waves	
7	Pure Water/ Neutral_____	
7.5	Blood	*weak alkaline*
8.5	Shampoo/Hand soap	
9.5	Ammonium Thio Perm	
10	Semi-permanent color	

10.0-13	Sodium Hydroxide (relaxer)
10.5	Permanent color/Tints/Toners
12.0	Bleach Boosters/Ammonia
14	Depilatory *strong alkaline*

Chemical Hair Relaxing

Chemical hair relaxing is the process of permanently breaking the S-bonds in the hair to get the hair to a permanently straightened condition. Some types of chemical straighteners are Sodium Hydroxide, and Calcium Hydroxide. There are two processes in chemical hair relaxing, **Virgin** and **Retouch.** First let's define the two. A **retouch** is applying a chemical to the new-growth area only. This procedure is used when a relaxer is already in the hair and the new hair needs to be straightened as it grows out from the scalp. A

virgin relaxer is when the hair has never had a relaxer, or when returning to a relaxer from a natural or non-chemical style. There are some things that you need to know if you are applying a relaxer yourself. I will give you some tips to help your next service be a success. But, if at all possible, leave any chemical services to a licensed professional, especially permanent color. Be sure to select the correct strength of relaxer for your hair texture and type. If you have hair that is colored or highlighted, make absolute sure that you are using only a color-treated or mild relaxer, and wait two week and at least one shampoo to allow for proper conditioning. If you are considering getting permanent color, change the strength of relaxer months prior to your color service to prepare for the color process. The reason is if you have a regular strength or super relaxer already and your hair and apply a permanent haircolor or bleach product to your hair on top of that relaxer, then the hair could break immediately. As a result, when the hair is shampooed, the hair will go right down the drain.

If you must apply your own relaxer, here are some tips.

Retouch Tips

#1 Check for any abrasions or scalp irritations; Do not proceed if any are present.

#2 Start by selecting the correct relaxer strength for your hair type

#3 Use gloves

#4 Apply a protective base on the scalp and around the hairline and ears to prevent burns or irritation.

#5 Avoid overlapping onto hair that has already been relaxed; use a cream to avoid over-processing pre-relaxed hair

#6 Part hair in four sections and start in the most resistant area. DO NOT apply around the hairline first. Hairline areas are the weakest areas on the head though you may not think so. Relaxing these areas first can result in thinning or breakage around the hairline, over time. Apply to the hairline last.

#7 Be careful not to spread the relaxer over hair that has already been relaxed, over time this weakens the hair causing the hair to break. The correct procedure is to apply the relaxer to the hair and gently smooth with the back of the comb or with the finger. Avoid excessive pulling or stretching while relaxing. Remember, the relaxer is a strong chemical and the product has the ability to soften the hair without excessive stretching or combing.

#8 after hair is relaxed, rinse thoroughly, and then follow the manufacturer's directions. Pay close attention, that there is no relaxer left in the hair especially in the nape and top area if you are relaxing your own hair. Sometimes manufacturers will include a color coded shampoo that will turn the shampoo a pinkish color to let you know there is still relaxer in the hair. If there is, repeat the shampoo procedure until the shampoo shows no signs of pink.

#9 In order to ensure that the relaxer is properly rinsed from the hair, make sure that your water is under pressure. This pressure helps ensure that the water will reach the scalp area, where the relaxer has been placed, to remove all traces of the relaxer.

WARNING! If any relaxer is left in the hair, the hair will break even after the hair is dried and styled. If your water doesn't have enough pressure, go to a licensed professional. Trust me, you would rather pay for a professional to render the services rather than pay for treatments to fix a potential problem, as they can be very costly.

#10 Again, follow manufacturer's instructions!!
#11 Use a Neutralizing shampoo after relaxer, and never use a neutralizing shampoo for a basic

shampoo. Neutralizing shampoo is used to lower the pH of the hair and to stop the action of the relaxer.

#12 Proceed with suggested conditioner, or treatment, process and style as desired.

Virgin Relaxer tips

#1 follow steps 1-4 of previous section.

#2 when doing a virgin relaxer, Do Not apply relaxer directly to the new-growth area first. The full length of the hair must be straightened before it is applied to the new growth area and hair ends. To do so will result in the hair being under-processed because the full length of the hair will not have time to process before discomfort may be felt on the scalp.

#3 Begin the relaxer about ½-inch to 1 inch from the scalp and up to ½ inch from the ends. Once the relaxer has been applied in this manner throughout all four sections, began applying relaxer to the new-growth area throughout all sections. Then began smoothing and applying to the ends. Once hair is sufficiently relaxed or straightened, rinse relaxer thoroughly, shampoo and follow manufacturer's directions. Style as desired.

Relaxer Selection Chart

Color Treated or Mild Relaxer	Regular/Normal Relaxer	Super/Resistant Relaxer
Color Treated Highlighted Bleached Frosted Permanent color Lightened or Fine Hair	Normal or Med. Textured hair	Coarse/thick Resistant gray hair

Natural Hair Styling

In today's society, there are lots of African Americans making the choice to go natural. There are lots of options for natural hairstyling. These options include: braids, knots, twist, dread locks, afro, or press and curl, to name a few. One important factor is to make sure you give proper care to the hair and scalp. When you decide to go natural, it is very important that the hair is given as much conditioning as possible. Because natural hair has a tendency to be dry, you need to make sure that you select products that contain moisturizers for your hair and scalp. Since natural hair is so popular, there are a host of manufacturers with lines specifically for natural hair. These include scalp oils or sprays for dry, flaky or itchy scalp, shampoos, conditioners, moisturizers, sheens and glosses, to name a few. Take advantage of these products as they have everything you need for your choice of styling. Make sure that you take the necessary steps to keep the hair and scalp clean. Do not leave the hair up for extensive periods of time without cleansing the scalp and hair, to do so may result in disorders of the scalp, not to mention an odor in the hair. The hair and scalp must be cleansed.

Since natural hair is much stronger than relaxed hair, you have more options for things such as permanent color. You may choose to go blonde or platinum, as long as it accentuates your complexion or eye color. Seek a professional for this type of coloring since no hair is beyond being damaged.

Natural hair can be pressed, flat ironed or just worn in an afro. If you choose to flat iron or press your hair, make sure you use a heat protector, like curling wax, to protect from heat styling. Also, choose a ceramic flat iron which will prevent you from burning the hair from the outside of the strands. This flat iron is a healthier choice than your standard flat iron. If you are using a flat iron, you may need to use a small pressing comb for your edges as the flat iron may not give you the straightness around the edges.

WARNING!! Never get a relaxer before braiding as it may cause breakage. The natural hair is much stronger than hair that has been relaxed. A relaxer takes away some of the hair's strength when it is straightened. I know you would like to have your "edges" straight, but when hair is braided, it is pulled so tightly that it will give the appearance that the hair is already straightened.

WARNING 2!!!!! Please don't allow anyone to put glue on your hair, when getting braids (nail glue, super glue etc.) to camouflage where the natural hair ends and the braided or added hair begins. This may sound crazy, but I know from experience that this happens. I had to cut off just about all of my client's hair. Why? Because she let an unlicensed person braid her hair and she put some type of glue on her hair to keep the hair from coming loose. The glue melted the fibers of the hair together and could not come out. So I had only one option, cut it off beyond the point of the glue. This resulted in the client getting a 2 inch cut from having a shoulder-length bob.

NOTE: Find an experienced and licensed braider if a braided style is desired.   Cheaper is not always better.

Extensions, Weave, Tracks

The healthiest way to get extensions or tracks is to have the natural hair braided and have the extensions sewn in. Another way is to have someone attach the extensions or tracks to a stocking cap, cut, and style and wear the stocking cap as you would a wig. These are popular and fashionable.

If you must get the extensions applied using glue, allow the stylist to remove them instead of removing them yourself. There are products on the market that helps soften the glue and makes removal easier and causes less damage to the hair. Excessive pulling of the tracks will increase the chances of loosing more hair and destroying the papilla. Remember, if the papilla is destroyed, the hair will not grow back. If you notice thinning after using extensions, avoid another application until the hair has been properly treated and the condition of the hair improves. If you have substantial damage and thinning, stop using extensions or weave, Altogether. The continued use of tracks or extensions in this case will eventually result in extensive thinning that can sometimes become permanent. Go to a licensed stylist who can suggest a cut or style that will accentuate your features while down playing thinning. In my opinion, it is easier to style and cut the hair if the damage is in the nape area as you can get a short pixie or tapered style. However, if the damage or thinning is in the front, top (crown) or back it is more difficult to create a style because you must have enough hair to cover thinning areas unless you choose to be cut down to an afro. Ultimately, if you continue to get extensions glued in when the hair and scalp shows damage, you could destroy any future chances of the hair returning back to its normal state. I can't stress enough that if the papilla is destroyed, the hair will not grow back. Without hair, where will you glue your extensions?

Let's face it, we have enough to contend with in stress, illnesses, medications, hormone imbalances, hereditary issues etc. without adding insult to injury.

Permanent Waving

The main active ingredient used in alkaline permanents is **Ammonium Thioglycolate ("thio")**. The pH of alkaline waving solution generally ranges from 8.2-9.6 depending on the amount of ammonia. Alkaline perms soften and swell the cuticle layer allowing the solution to penetrate faster than acid-balanced solutions. Some alkaline perms can be wrapped with either water or waving lotion and gives a strong curl pattern.

Glyceryl Monothioglycolate is the main active ingredient in Acid-balanced perms. These perms have a pH of 4.5-6.5. An acid-balanced perm lowers the pH and usually gives a softer curl, and is gentler on the hair. However, they require longer processing time usually with heat for curl development. Heat may be activated chemically, within the product which is called *exothermic* or by a hooded dryer called *endothermic*.

Permanent wave solution reforms or rearranges the S-Bonds to allow the hair to take the shape of the rod used to reach the desired curl pattern.   A permanent wave is applied to add curl to straight hair.   Some alkaline perms may either be wrapped with wave solution or wrapped with water when rodded.

Always follow manufacturer's directions. Below is a general guideline used to select the perm that is right for you. Keep in mind that there are alkaline formulas for bleached hair as well as acid-balanced formulas for resistant hair. As I stated earlier, seek a licensed professional when chemical services are desired.

Permanent Wave Selection

Chart

Hair Texture	**Perm to Select**
Coarse Resistant	Alkaline lotion wrap or alkaline water wrap
Fine, Resistant	Alkaline lotion wrap or alkaline water wrap
Normal	Alkaline water wrap or acid-balanced
Normal, Porous	Alkaline water wrap or acid-balanced
Normal, Delicate	Acid-balanced
Tinted, Non-porous	Alkaline water wrap or acid-balanced
Tinted, Porous	Acid-balanced
Highlighted, Frosted/bleached	Acid-balanced

Alkaline Perms   Acid Perms

Alkaline Perms	Acid Perms
Stronger curl pattern wrapped with lotion	Weaker curl pattern
Process faster	Process slower
Room temp. processing	Requires Endothermic or exothermic heat
Use when clients curls easily relaxes or don't hold	Use on hair that is delicate, fragile or color-treated

*Chart by: sallybeauty.com

*Perms that are lotion wrapped usually produces stronger curls than water wrapped perms. Lotion wrapped is using the permanent waving solution to wrap or rod the hair for pre-softening resistant hair. Once the hair is rodded, the remaining solution is applied to the entire head.

Choosing the Right Shampoo

This may seem like a simple task, but the truth of the matter is that there are lots of people using the wrong shampoos. Shampoo should be selected according to the hair's condition and type. I will explain the main types of shampoos and what they should be used for.

Dry Shampoo-designed for client confined to bed, or client's health does not permit a wet shampoo. It cleans hair without water. When sprayed directly onto hair, dry shampoo penetrates the hair absorbing dirt and hair products. When brushed out, the dry shampoo takes all these impurities with it leaving clean hair. Do not use with a chemical service.

Anti-Dandruff Shampoo-is a medicated shampoo used to control itching and flaking associated with dandruff, dermatitis, seborrhea and scalp psoriasis.

Anti-Frizz Shampoo- used to control frizz or wiry, unruly hair. It restores moisture to hair and prevents and smoothes frizz.

Clarifying Shampoo- used to remove product build-up, medication and chlorine or minerals from showers and pools. Always come back with a moisturizer or hydrating conditioner afterwards.

Thickening or Volumizing Shampoo-maximizes thickness, strength and adds volume. The cortex is infused with nutrients and moisture to strengthen and expand the diameter of each hair strand.

Color Shampoo-used to enhance or revitalize color treated hair and is available in a variety of shades.

Shampoos for thinning hair- These types of shampoos are therapeutic and promotes circulation which in turn stimulates hair follicles, creating a cleaner, healthier scalp to encourage new hair growth. Some of these are used to detoxify and clear the scalp from debris and DHT (dihydrotestosterone). DHT interrupts the hair growth cycle constricting the blood supply, oxygen and nutrients of the hair follicle.

Gray Hair Shampoo- Used to remove yellowish tinge from hair to enhance white or gray hair.

Damaged Hair Shampoo- Used to cleanse damaged hair, restores shine, and strengthens the hair. It also normalizes the pH.

Moisturizing/Hydrating Shampoo- Softens and adds shine, restores moisture to dry or extremely dry hair.

<u>Conditioning Shampoo</u>- Shampoo with a conditioner in it. They may contain conditioning agents such as: Protein, dimethicone, biotin, oleyl alcohol, cocoamphocarboxyglycinate.

Choosing the Right Conditioner

As there are many types of shampoos for many problems or needs, there are also conditioners. There are full lines of products available for your hair needs. As a rule of thumb, try to use the same line of products for your hair care problems or needs as they were designed to work in sync with one another. If your hair is thinning, stick to one line of products all for "thinning hair". The best conditioner is only a temporary remedy for problem or damaged hair. It cannot "heal", damaged hair, nor can it improve the quality or the new hair growth. Heredity, Health, and Diet control the texture and structure of the hair. However, it is valuable because it can minimize the damage during a service and it can restore lusture, shine, manageability, and strength while the damaged hair grows long enough to be cut off and replaced by new hair. Most conditioners fall in the pH range of 3.5 to 6.0; therefore they have the ability to restore the pH balance after an alkaline chemical treatment.

The main types of conditioners are: Instant Conditioners, Moisturizers, Reconstructors/Protein Conditioners and Packs.

Instant conditioners may remain on the hair from 1-5 minutes or may be a leave-in containing humectants to improve the appearance of dry brittle hair. Humectants are chemical compouds that absorbs and hold moisture from the hair and temporarily locks in moisture. Some ingredients are: Cetyl alcohol and stearyl alcohol, which works as a pearlizing agent and lubricates to leave hair with a glossy finish; Lanolin/Sheep oil for fine hair, because of molecular weight, and Silicone oils such as simethicone and dimethicone for finishing sheen.

Moisturizers contain small molecules which enable the conditioner to penetrate the layers of the hair. Some may incorporate heat and others may not. Other conditioners contain large molecules that are not capable of penetrating the hair shaft. These are generally conditioners that detangle, which weigh hair down and make hair easier to comb. Quats are included in moisturizers. Stearatkonium chloride is also used in moisturizers to counteract the drying affects of anionic detergents and chemical treatments.

Protein /Reconstructors are polymers, many units, composed of combinations of any of

23 amino acids used to recondition damaged hair. These are used to increase tensile strength of hair and to temporarily close split ends. They replace keratin that has been lost. They also improve texture, equalize porosity and increase elasticity. However, these should not be used immediately after a chemical treatment, because they can alter freshly completed and desirable rearrangement of protein bonds after a permanent wave, relaxer or hair coloring.

Packs are chemical mixtures of concentrated protein in the heavy cream base of a moisturizer. They penetrate several cuticle layers.

Conditioners for hair thinning are products that contain ingredients used to stimulate the scalp causing blood to circulate, to nourish the hair, and to promote growth. It usually gives a tingling sensation on the scalp.

Styling Agent/Products

Last but not least, I will give you a brief overview of styling agents used to protection the hair and finish the style.

Curling Wax- Used to protect hair from heat styling; Marcel irons, flat irons, blow drying, etc.

Oil Sheen- imparts shine to hair; may be used before, during or after styling.

Spritz-Used to hold style in place, or sometimes used while curling with heat. Spritz comes in a variety of holding power. With soft-hold spritz, the hair can still be combed after it is applied. Hard/firm hold spritz should not be combed. This type freezes the style in place and to comb it can cause damage to the hair.

Spray Gloss or Liquid Gloss – A clear gloss in spray or liquid form used to add shine. Most contain silicone which helps prevent frizz.

Holding Spray-Hairspray used to hold style in place. This is usually a finishing product.

Humidity Resistant-Used to prevent frizziness and split ends; provides hold with UV protectants.

Medicated Scalp Oil-Relieves itchiness and dryness of the scalp while adding shine and moisture. They may contain anti-fungal and anti-bacterial agents. These ingredients kill fungus that may clog the hair follicle that may prevent or slow down hair growth.

Pomades- used to add definition to a style such as spikes. Also adds texture.

Gels- Used to add hold, or to mold the hair to the head to prepare for further styling. Try to use gel that contains little or no alcohol.

Volumizing Styling Aids- Usually applied to the scalp area to add lift and volume.

Final Thought

As with any other problems or issues you may be experiencing, be sure to consult a medical professional or a licensed hairstylist for services or diagnosis. This book is for information purposes and also may serve as a guide to help give insight to some common problems or concerns you may have about hair care or hair thinning.

I hope you find this book useful to you and I wish you the best. You may send comments or emails to iristus@yahoo.com. May God Bless.

Resources

* www.Webmd.com/skin-problems-and-treatments/hair-loss/drug-induced-hairloss

* WebMD Medical Reference from the American Hair Loss Association

* Mary Sheen's Fighting Hair Loss

* www.Haircoloringtips.com

* www.Exploratorium.edu

* International Trichology Consultants

* www.pg.com

* hairandscalp.com

* sallybeauty.com

* combat-hair-loss.co.uk

* restorationhair.com

* Milady's Standard Textbook of Cosmetology

* Reba Roy

Notes

Notes

_____

_____

_____

_____

_____

_____

_____

_____

_____

_____

_____

_____

_____

_____

_____

_____

9 780615 205601